Choi

A Step Towards The Altar

Discover How To Choose A Mate And The Relevance of Counselling Before You Say "I Do"

William And Rev. Mrs Dorothy Appiah

EQUIPPED FOR SUSTAINABLE

MARRIAGE - BOOKS

Choice & Courtship: A Step Towards The Altar

Discover How To Choose A Mate And The Relevance of Counselling Before You Say "I Do"

sought. This book is not intended for use as a source of legal or accounting advice. Any reference to any person or business whether living or dead is purely coincidental.

The House of Change,
Christian Counselling, Coaching and Advocacy Centre
Unit 7 Excalibur Works,
13 Argall Avenue
Argall Industrial Estates
E10 7QE, London, UK

ISBN: 978-1-910894-03-3

Copies are available at special rates for bulk orders. Contact The House of Change,
Email: **AdminPublishing@TheHouseOfChange.com**
Website: www.TheHouseOfChange.com

❀ "Me ware wo."- "I shall marry you". Akan, Adinkra symbol of commitment, perseverance. From the expression "No one rushes into the job of mixing the concrete for building the house of marriage.

✺ "Mmere dane" - "Time changes ". Symbol of change, life's dynamics By G. F. Kojo Arthur , Cloth As Metaphor: (Re)reading the adinkra cloth symbols of the Akan of Ghana. Accra: Cefiks Publications, 2001.

Words of wisdom

"Everyone who hears these words of mine and does them will be like a wise man who built his house upon the rock; and the rain fell, and the floods came, and the winds blew and beat upon the house, but it did not fall, because it had been founded on a rock.

And everyone who hears these words of mine and does not do them will be like a foolish man who built his house upon the sand; and the rain fell, and the floods came, and the winds blew and beat against that house, and it fell; and great was the fall of it".

Jesus Christ of Nazareth
Matthew 7:24-27

EQUIPPED FOR SUSTAINABLE MAR-
RIAGE BOOKS

From

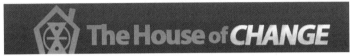

About the Authors

William & Rev. Mrs Dorothy Appiah are Christian Counsellors and Life Breakthrough Coaches. William and Dorothy have been counselling individuals and couples for over a decade. They do face to face counselling as well as group counselling. They also provide their services to some clients via Skype, phone and email. They have special skills and interests in Personal development and Relationship Coaching and are also FOCCUS Inc, USA, trained in marriage preparation inventory.

William is a Christian Author and a Publisher. He is a Journalist, Public Relations and Communications specialist. He is also an Environmentalist by profession as well as Stakeholder Relations and Networking expert.

He obtained his B.A (Hons) degree and MSc. in Environmental Policy from the University of Ghana, Legon and University of London, UK. He also has a Graduate Diploma in Communication Studies from the School of Communications, University of Ghana. He is also an Infopreneur, Social Media Expert, Internet Marketer and Public Speaker on Sustainable Marriages and Personal Development.

Rev. Dorothy is a Minister of God. She is a public speaker on building and sustaining marriages, Women issues and a Trainer in Christian Marriage Counselling for Churches. Her special calling is in teaching the Word of God, Prayer and Women Empowerment and Development issues. She is a well-known Christian Marriage Counsellor, a Life Breakthrough Coach and a Motivational Speaker. Rev. Dorothy is also a specialist in talking to Men Groups about women and Women Groups about men. She is a member of Christian Coaching Alliance, USA, a network of Christian life and leadership coaches worldwide. She is the founder of Minister Dorothy's Ministries For Women Empowerment. She is also the Coordinator, of SaferHaven, a network of African Pastors wives for the Advancement of Ministry worldwide.

The couple are founders of The House of Change, a Christian Counselling, Life Breakthrough Coaching and Advocacy Centre and Authors and Publishers of Equipped for Sustainable Marriage books. They are members of Praise Harvest Community Church (Part of Praise Harvest International Ministries), U.K. They have been married for over twenty five years and have three children: Jesse, Sean and William.

PURPOSE

My purpose is that they may be encouraged in heart and united in love, so that they may have full riches of complete understanding, in order that they may know the mystery of God, namely Christ, in whom are hidden all the treasures of wisdom and knowledge.

—Colossians. 2:3,4

FOOD FOR THOUGHT

"To those who have ears, let them hear. We are coming from your future - with 25 years of a happy, sustainable and fulfilled marriage - into your present to hold your hand, inform and guide you to where you are planning to go - marriage".

—William and Rev Mrs Dorothy Appiah

Dedication

This book is dedicated to our three sons, Jesse, Sean and William, who asked insightful and thought provoking questions and inspired us to complete this book.

It is also dedicated to all Christians in Relationships.

"So others may enjoy a happy, sustainable and fulfilled relationships."

We are grateful to God Almighty who gave us the wisdom to complete this book. Glory be to His name.

Contents

Acknowledgement

A very big thank you goes to all those who provided information and assistance while we were writing this book. Special thanks to Pastor Moses Asare, Head Pastor of Praise Harvest Community Church, London, and his wife Nana Agyemang, for their spiritual support, advice and information.

Our special thanks also go to Serwaa Adomako for her time, resources and technical support and her belief that this book can be published.

Benjamin Agyemang, a Lecturer and consultant, and Rev Dr Solomon Brobbey, proved beyond doubt that they are our good friends.

Our gratitude also goes to Allan and Donna Goerz, renowned Marriage Counsellors, who provided much training and information during the early years.

Our new found "angel", Lesley Spurrel, for her editing, proof reading and invaluable suggestions. We are very grateful.

Special thanks to Rev. Joseph Brako, Praise Harvest

William And Rev. Mrs Dorothy Appiah

Community Church, South London, and his dear wife Nana Akua, for their belief that it is possible to write and publish this book,

Last but not least is my brother, Kwasi Aboagye-Atta, and his dear wife, Patricia. for their words of encouragement, proof reading, time and making us believe that it is possible to produce this book.

Introduction

Marriage is for life. Once you have decided to be part of the institution, you must ensure you succeed. We decided to write about the basics for choosing a partner, courtship and finally marriage in order to enlighten readers on what they needed to know before plunging into it. Some people have described the institution of marriage as a life sentence; once you are in it, you must sustain it.

Most of the time, young people have no information, knowledge or understanding of what they will face. Several young people have entered into marriage in ignorance only to find out that "not everything that glitters is gold".

We have tried to provide a range of information from a personal perspective, from the experts and also from the Bible. We have had our own experiences regarding these issues. Our interest in marriage counselling for the last decade has opened our eyes to the fact that with a proper foundation, people can sustain their marriage, especially when the wind of change blows.

We married when we were mature. We were determined to make the marriage work. Our determination led us to seek more knowledge and information. We believe that this book, which is infused with our experiences, will help you during your dating and courtship and provide you with the much-needed information. Our Christian beliefs have contributed to our happy and sustainable marriage for over 25 years. It is our considered view that the biblical statement, "we should not be unequally yoked with unbelievers" should be taken seriously in your search for a partner.

In all issues concerning relationships, we must be guided by the word of God. He is the one who instituted marriage and therefore has all the answers. We need to pray constantly in our search for partners and for our marriage. In all things, ask for wisdom from God. He alone can provide you with it in abundance.

Lastly, seek counselling. It is a sign of strength. Further knowledge, in addition to that which you already have, will ensure that you enjoy a happy lasting marriage in the future. Whilst we are aware that good marriages start long before the premarital counselling, a counsellor is necessary to help you through the changes you will be facing. Therefore, we have included valuable information to explain what premarital counselling is, the goals, the reasons for choosing pre-marital counselling as well as information on when to begin the counselling.

Marriage can be happy and fulfilling but also involves effort, risk, and times of difficulty and disappointment. These are not easy experiences. When you have a better foundation and the storms of life hit your marriage, your anchor will hold. When things seem to go wrong and you have the right partner, the strong foundation you have laid will help you through. You can work through the challenges and problems in life with a compatible partner with far greater success than with someone who was the wrong choice.

Trust God for a happy marriage. He knows best.

CHAPTER 1

MATE SELECTION: CHOOSING A SUITABLE PARTNER

Knowledge and Information

The lack of accurate knowledge about relationships before marriage is one of the main causes of divorce. "The fear of the Lord is the beginning of wisdom, but fools despise wisdom and discipline. Proverbs 1: 7. You need knowledge to be able to make the right choice. Divorce is now a common phenomenon even within Christian circles, though it is not encouraged. Many believers, including Pastors and Christian leaders, have divorced after years of marriage. The oath "for better or for worse, until death do us part" is no longer seen as sacred and therefore couples are prepared to end whatever marriage covenant they have made when they are no longer "in love" with each other.

Christians should be wiser and many do seek information from their Pastors, friends, parents and marriage counsellors before making the final choice of a partner, however when people are already in love and are emotionally connected, it is sometimes too late to advise them. To them, love is a feeling and therefore they are not able to translate it into words. They are unable to explain what is happening to them once they are emotionally involved.

It is important that information is given and preventative blocks put in place before the individuals choose their prospective mates. With appropriate advice and education, it is less difficult to remove the unhealthy attitudes and behaviours that may lead to the unwise selection of a marriage partner. "Facts about mate selection tend to lose significance and influence after one has fallen in love. If facts and warnings can be given before emotional bonds are allowed to develop, it seems more likely that error will be avoided and potentially harmful involvements may be resisted" noted Gary Collins, Author and a Christian Counsellor.

We are of the considered opinion that people armed with accurate knowledge and information before marriage have a better chance of succeeding in their relationship. You need to be physically, spiritually and psychologically prepared for marriage. This is the only way to prevent the widespread divorces taking place in society today.

Scriptures

The Bible is very clear on who to marry, but says very little about mate selection. Jesus Christ approved marriages and even participated in some. His first miracle of turning water into wine occurred at a wedding ceremony. Some scholars believe that this silence, within the scriptures, may reflect the fact that during biblical times, choosing a mate was not the couple's responsibility; it was the responsibility of the parents.

The Bible's guideline is straightforward. Believers are only to marry believers. Therefore, a Christian should not marry a non-Christian. "Don't team up with those who are unbelievers. How can goodness be a partner with wickedness? How can light live with darkness?" 2 Cor. 6:14. A similar idea is expressed in 1 Corinthians and specifically applied to marriage when Paul says that an unmarried woman is free to marry whomever she wishes but only if the marriage is acceptable to the Lord. This clearly implies that she must marry a fellow believer.

Neil Warren in his book, *Finding the love of your life,* said; "Your choice of whom to marry is more crucial than everything else combined you will ever do to make your marriage succeed."

He also said – outside of your commitment to Christ, marriage is the most important commitment a human being can make

The bible advises singles not to be equally yoked with unbelievers. This passage is sometimes seen as an unfair statement to many, especially when they think or believe they are in love, usually, when the heart flatters and the mind stops working.

This advice is somehow treated lightly, especially when individuals are choosing a life partner. The reason is that whatever you are yoked with, you share its weight. While the believer's yoke is made light in Christ, that of the unbeliever is not so. The unbeliever thus brings a burden which your carrying capacity cannot cope. This may have serious effects on your marriage in future.

It is significant to note that the unbeliever is still in the pit and needs to be pulled out. You will always need a greater force to pull them out.

Another important point is that, your body is the temple of God and need to be kept holy. You cannot give what has been kept holy to just any person. This is because if the person is an unbeliever, he or she may end up contaminating you spiritually.

Furthermore, experience has shown that unbelievers do not respect the values, culture and traditions of Christianity. In our several years of counselling, some of the issues of conflict in relationships centre on misunderstanding of one's Christian values. The unbeliever is well rooted and grounded in his ways so the more you grow in your Christian walk the more you move away from your partner.

This will also affect the way your children will be brought up; in the Lord or in worldly ways or the beliefs of your partner.

It is, however, very surprising how many believers can rationalise their choice to marry an unbeliever by giving all sorts of excuses. Twenty years ago, we witnessed the marriage of a lady friend, whom we knew from the University, to "Mr Right" at the Registry Office. The lady was a believer, while the man was not. She was so madly in love that any reference to the fact that the man was an unbeliever was bound to upset her. Against their better judgement, and after much persuasion, the parents gave in to their daughter's wishes.

Several years later, the couple had children. The man forbade the woman to take the children to church despite the fact that they had agreed on this issue prior to the marriage. The children were not baptised and were given names which became a severe problem and an embarrassment for the wife. She could not mention her own children's names in public and among her friends. Eventually, the couple divorced.

Divine Guidance

Divine Guidance is the best and preferred option. Several Biblical passages teach that believers can expect divine leading, even though this may not come in dramatic or seemingly miraculous ways. God speaks to each and everyone in different ways. Be attentive the spirit of the Lord within you. Christians are divided over the issue of whether God has only one choice for a person who is seeking a life partner. It is difficult to find Biblical support for the idea that in the entire universe, God has only one person for each of us, that the identity of this person will be revealed in time, and that life will be unhappy if you marry someone else. Clearly, 1 Corinthians 7 teaches that marriage and remaining single are both acceptable to God and the choice of a mate is governed only by the requirement that Christians must marry Christians. Beyond that, it would appear that a Christian is free to choose a marriage partner based on his or her own careful reflection and the thoughtful input of other people, including parents or a trusted Christian counsellor.

Other Considerations

Being a Christian is not a guarantee for compatibility in marriage. There are other factors which need to be taken into consideration. These are enumerated in this book.

However, there are also two important issues that need to be taken into consideration. The first is the vision of the man as well as each other's plans for the future. You cannot simply just follow someone whose future plans and vision you don't know. We believe that it is in your own interest to find out the future plans.

The second important issue is about sex. We always try to find out whether they are attracted to each other physically. It is natural to think about sex. Pause and think about what you find attractive about your partner. Is it the face, teeth, breadth, how clean the person is, his orher dressing? It is vital to make and give complimentary remarks. And is there some sexual attraction between the two of you? In most cases, the couples have not thought about sex. They even do not talk about it. They have left it until after the marriage. Unfortunately, they get a rude shock of their lives when after the marriage, they realise that their sex life is frustrating and not as they expected.

Why Choose a Partner?

In society today, people get married because they are in love. But love and feelings can be all too confusing and vague. Some Christian writers explains appropriately that, to fall in love is to feel elated, an exciting closeness and intimacy with another person of the opposite sex. But this emotional high does not last forever.

For deep love to persist and grow there must be a giving, other centred relationship similar to that described in 1 Corinthians 13. Gary Collins explains that, "it may be that for most people, deep and secure love comes after marriage. To grow in love is to involve oneself deliberately in acts of giving and caring. A feeling of being in love is not, in itself, a solid basis for marriage and, equally, the fact that "we don't love each other anymore" is not a valid basis for divorce.

In practical terms however, being in love has a place in choosing a life partner, but should not be the only basis. There are people who cannot leave with someone who they do not have at least an attraction for, in the initial place even before they begin to work at those qualities that root, grow and build that initial attraction.

The short answer to why we should choose a marriage partner is ultimately because God created us male and female, and declared, in his word, that marriage is honourable.

On Our way to London for one of our monthly seminars, we heard this short story on one of London's radio stations: Two men were talking;

1st man: I got married because I was tired of eating out, cleaning the house, doing the laundry & wearing shabby clothes.

2nd Man: Amazing, I just got divorced for the very same reasons.

The moral of the story is whether you have examined why you want to get married? Do not get married for all the wrong reasons.

Reasons

In the society today, people marry for reasons other than love and emotions. Their reasons may be diverse, but often centre on the idea of needs. Gary Collins points out that, marriage meets the need for:

- Mutual companionship

- Security

- Support

- Intimacy

- Friendship

- Sexual fulfilment

- Premarital pregnancy

- Social pressure from friends or parents.

- The desire to escape from an unhappy home environment

- The fear that one will be left alone

- A compulsion to rescue some unfortunate single person.

- Rebellion

- Escape

- Loneliness

- Physical pressure

He also notes that "Each of these reasons for marriage meets some need, although none in itself can be the basis for a mature and stable relationship".

Financial Reasons

An interesting reason for marriage, that has existed since the institution began, comes down to money. Due to circumstances such as poverty, the background of those concerned and the need to maintain class, there are people who purposely seek out partners with money. Another reason is the desire to be among the rich at any cost. Furthermore, there are families who are determined to maintain the status quo by ensuring that their children do not marry from outside their networks or social circles. Some families think, rightly or wrongly, that they have struggled for their wealth and therefore, will not accept "gold-diggers".

Marrying because your partner has a lot of money is not a good reason unless you are compatible in more fundamental ways. This is a basic truth. You may indeed succeed in marrying your partner, but soon the novelty of marrying a very rich person will wear off and the real nature of the relationship will gradually reveal itself.

In the same way, marrying a partner because of his or her material possessions, for example, a car, is also not a firm basis for the marriage and will not allow the relationship to weather the storms of life and time. Some people fall in love with 'the car' belonging to an individual rather than the owner. Most of us have heard such stories. One question we always ask is whether the marriage would end once the symbolic car is involved in an accident, destroyed, or out of fashion. We still don't have an answer.

H/C

Words of wisdom

His left hand is under my head,
And his right hand embraces me.
I charge you, O daughters of Jerusalem,
By the gazelles or by the does of the field,
Do not stir up nor awaken love
Until it pleases.

—Song of Solomon 2: 6-7

CHAPTER 2

ROMANCE AND MATE SEARCH

Romantic Excitement

Does romance affect the search for a partner? Some people agree it does. According to Sarah Litvinoff, Relate Marriage Expert, romantic love is wonderful. It is not simply a myth; it is also a real experience: dizzy, passionate, exciting and intoxicating. To be romantically in love is about the most thrilling thing that can happen to us. The myth is that this heightened romantic state is 'true' love, the best kind of love and more damaging still-that it can or should last.

Dr James Dobson, a well known expert in marriage counselling explained romantic love in his book, "What wives wish their husbands knew about women," that love is not simply a feeling of romantic excitement; it is more than a desire to marry a potential partner; it goes beyond intense sexual attraction; it exceeds the thrill at having "captured" a highly desirable social prize. These are emotions that are unleashed at first sight but they do not constitute love.

Dr Dobson explained further that "I wish the whole world knew that fact. These temporary feelings differ from love in that they place the spotlight on the one experiencing them. What is happening to me?! This is the most fantastic thing I have ever been through. I think I am in love!" You see, these emotions are selfish in the sense that that they are motivated by our gratification. They have to do with the new lover. Such a person has not fallen in love with another person; he has fallen in love with you! And there is an enormous difference between the two.... Real love, in contrast to popular belief, is an expression of the deepest appreciation for another human being; it is an intense awareness of his or her needs and longings – past, present and future. It is unselfish and giving and caring. And believe me friends, these are not behaviours one "falls" into at first sight as if tumbling into a ditch".

H. Norman Right disagrees and explains that romance is an important factor in choosing a mate. He explains, however, that it is important to distinguish between genuine love and romantic love. Romantic love has been labelled "cardiac-respiratory" love. This is love with an emphasis on excitement, thrills and palpitations of the heart. Some people react as if there were a lack of oxygen in the area. Ecstasy, daydreaming and a deep physical yearning are all indications of this malady. Not only is this type of love blind, it is also destructive. Neither the past nor the future is taken into consideration in evaluating the potential of the relationship.

But the question is whether romantic idealisations are so bad. The fact is that most people begin with romance, either romanticisation of the potential partner or the potential union. It is such a common and natural occurrence that we doubt a relationship can even begin without it.

H Norman Right explained further that "It is difficult to know how pervasive the romantic fallacy really is. I suspect that it creates the greatest havoc with high school seniors or the half of the population who are married before they are twenty years old. Nevertheless, even in a college or young adult population, one constantly finds, as a final criterion for marriage, the issue of being in love. This is due to the distortion, by the press, of the meaning of companionship within marriage, and by the cultural impact upon the last two or three generations. The result is that more serious and sober aspects of marital choice and marital expectations are not only neglected but also sometimes ridiculed".

Self-Marketing

Some researchers view the process of mate selection as an exercise in self-marketing. The reality is that individuals looking for a mate may present themselves and their attributes in as positive a light as possible, and they seek to find the best partner available for what they can offer in return. Consequently, if you are not able to market yourself effectively and efficiently, you may have all the potential but would pass unnoticed.

If individuals position themselves strategically, they will be in a better position to attract the mate of their choice. It is a case of being at the right place at the right time. There is nothing wrong with individuals making themselves visible to those they are interested in, but wisdom must be applied to the initial approach. Many people have missed out on individuals they were interested in dating. They were simply too shy to approach them and start a conversation. "Many people fail to strike when the opportunity presents itself." so goes the saying. People lose potential partners when the chance presents itself. They fail to capitalise when the opportunities are available. It is good to pray and seek for God's wisdom and guidance concerning a partner you wish to date, but timing is also important. You cannot delay for too long in case you lose out to another bolder person.

With some people, it is simply a question of a fear of failure. The fear of being rejected or the fear of what the other person might think about them discourages some from taking any action.

The world does not belong to the shy and mild person. It belongs to the bold, courageous and adventurous people, those who are prepared to go forward and take risks. Nothing ventured, nothing gained. This is the principle. You need to be confident and brave.

Where to Look for a Mate

If you know where to meet your ideal mate, then we believe that you may have overcome a very important constraint. However, this is not the case with most people. Several decades of research have confirmed that most people select mates from people who are of a similar age, education, social class, economic or income level, religion, race and place of residence. This is changing in this era of globalisation as both travel and cross-cultural communication become easier.

The reality, however is that, in looking for a mate, most people try to find someone who is of a similar background and social, religious and educational level.

Nowadays, it is even about class, whether they are of the same social standing. Within this broad category, the choice of a partner is narrowed by one's personal standards, parental approval or disapproval and by the single person's mental image of an ideal mate.

Most unmarried people go about their daily lives with some observant and watchful readiness to meet potential mates at seminars, conferences, school, church, and social gatherings who meet their mental image of the potential ideal partner.

They are alert to the fact that they may see or meet possible partners with whom they may strike up a casual friendship. Sometimes it may be work mates or neighbours or chance strangers or long time friends, on your way to or from work. This may later develop into a serious relationship.

The arrival of the Internet has also increased opportunities for finding potential mates, for example in the use of online mate-selection or 'dating' services. It is however, very important to apply wisdom and Godly principles in your search for a partner. Do not throw caution to the wind.

✿ Words of wisdom

To live is to choose. But to choose well, you must know who you are and what you stand for, where you want to go and why you want to get there.

—Kofi Annan
Former UN Secretary-General

CHAPTER 3

Choice: A Lifetime Decision Making

The Choices We Make

The choice we make in the search for a potential mate can ensure our future happiness or ruin our life and sometimes it is forever. In reality, choosing a mate is one of life's most important decisions. It involves emotions and passions, but it also needs to involve our brains, otherwise we will make foolish choices that we will later regret.

Those who marry *only* because of romance overlook the fact that partners need to possess certain credentials to be suitable to each other. Some make bad choices while others make good and well informed ones. But when you make a bad choice, you must be prepared to go with it. Thus "you have made your own bed and must be prepared to lie in it". The adage goes that "when you went fishing in the wide ocean that was the only golden fish you caught".

The reasons some people's choices prove favourable;

- Similar religious convictions; A Christian should not marry a non- Christian; that is what the Bible says. You must be wise and go out with a Christian in order to save yourself from emotional traumas later.

- Similar backgrounds; Mate selection is best when you share similar attributes such as values, age, socio-economic level, interests and education.

- Complementary needs; Meeting each other's needs are very advantageous and help to match and also harmonise the relationship.

- Good chemistry; when you flow emotionally and empathetically with the person, sometimes as if you have been friends or known each other for a long time. It has to do with feelings. You need this feeling to sustain the "spark" in your relationship.

Some people also choose unwisely. A friend said "it is always a bad mistake not to make the right choice"

Gary Collins explains that Social pressures, the influence of parents and friends, sexual urges or strong desires to get married are some of the influences urging people prematurely into unhealthy relationships. In addition, almost everybody brings expectations to their marriages, and these may face unpleasant challenges when reality sets in. Sometimes, single people look for a mate solely on the basis of what they can receive from marriage, but when married partners expect to receive without giving, they are heading for disappointment.

With a little reflection, most of us who have been in relationships for some time could list reasons why people make unwise choices. Tensions are likely to develop if a marriage partner is chosen primarily to

- Escape a difficult home situation

- Prove that one is an adult

- Rebel against parents or a former partner

- Escape the stigma of being single in society where it exists.

- Get an in-house sexual partner

- Bolster self esteem

- Improve social status

- "Find somebody to take care of me".

Future tensions can also arise due to:

- Wide age differences,

- Mental illness in one or both individuals

- Evidence of financial irresponsibility and insta-bility

- Substance abuse in one or both partners

- Differing religious beliefs,

- Individuals who have never dated anyone other than the intended mate.

What Exactly do you Want?

Within the broad category of social, religious and educational background and sometimes economic status, the choice of a partner is narrowed by one's personal standards, parental approval or disapproval and by the single person's mental image of an ideal mate.

What are your personal standards? What are the values you are looking for in a partner? What principles have you set for yourself? If you have not set any principles and values, what it means is that "everything goes". If you do not want an uneducated person, do not go in for one. If you do not want to marry a smoker, drug addict or a drunkard, do not make the mistake and choose one. The fact is that if you do not know what you want, you will not be able to see it and choose when it is even presented before you.

Does the person you want to marry meet your mental image? What is your mental view of a genuine future partner? What exactly are you looking for? If you are a woman and a real lady: Are you looking for a handsome or otherwise, tall, short, fat, slim, skinny, hairy or bald man among others? You will make the wrong choice if you don't know what you want. And what about a friendly, polite and strong willed man? The choice is yours. Think and make the right choice for life.

If you are a man and a real gentleman; what is your mental view of your future wife? Do you want a tall, short, slim, plump, fat or skinny lady? What is the size of lady you want including size zero? Is the front or the back side of the lady important to you? What about the hair? Do you want natural beauty? Nowadays, beauty can be found in the shop and can be bought at any price. And what about the inner beauty and the character of the lady? Are you looking for a virtuous woman? Think and make a good choice for life. Do not be too spiritual to close your eyes and mind.

Parental Expectations

It is a fact that whenever a new relationship begins, each partner has to bring the family into the equation. You all have family members whose opinion you respect and who have your best interest at heart. Their opinions are very important to you because of the role they play in your lives. These are the core members you need to speak with and introduce your partner to.

Your family may have high expectations of you due to your education, religious upbringing, background, social standing and other intangibles. Therefore, when you present your prince charming or beautiful princess and it does not meet their expectation, it becomes a bitter pill to swallow. Mothers especially, always pray and hope that their children will bring home the best mate that will meet their expectations. They believe that because they gave birth to you and have nurtured you from infancy, they know the type of person who will be suitable for you. For that reason, they are always on the look out. If your choice does not meet their set standard and mental image, you may be in for a faulty start in your relationship.

Jack, a young man had a relationship with Yvonne. The lady was well educated and had a Master's degree from a British University and a good job. Jack was well known to the parents. However, with time, cracks developed between them because the parents began to find faults with Jack. The main problem was that Jack's education was not to Yvonne's standard and he could not match their social standing. The parents thought their daughter deserved better.

One day, after running errands for Yvonne's family, Jack forgot his house keys at Yvonne's family house. The parent's were not pleased with the fact that a man of his stature could forget his keys. To them, that was a clear sign of irresponsibility, because keys are used to open doors and are treasured possessions which should never be left anywhere. It has deeper symbolic meanings for them. Though Jack and Yvonne are from the same country and have similar traditional background, that fact was not important at this stage since the boy had behaved irresponsibly. Their culture and traditional norms stipulates that if you loose something which is so dear to your heart and living such as your house key, that is a sure sign of irresponsibility. The parents therefore, saw Jack as an irresponsible boy and therefore discouraged their daughter from bringing him home. On the other hand, the parents encouraged the daughter to move on with her life, go ahead and search for a responsible man who can take care of her. At the end of the story, the relationship broke down due mainly to parental influence. Yvonne is currently married.

Sometimes, the writings would be on the wall in bold letters that the relationship would not last due to the fact that the partners are a mismatch. The parents would point them out, but the fact that both partners attend the same church and are somehow living to meet the expectations of the members, even when they see and read the signs on the wall, they would ignore them.

Some church members also ignorantly think that so far as they have mentioned to the Pastor of their Church that they are going out, they are bound to get married at any cost. This is far from the truth. You are not married. Therefore, when you think you are no more interested in each other, the honourable thing is to end the relationship and inform your pastor as a matter of courtesy. Live the life for yourself and do not be pressurised to live your life to suite others. Never live your personal life to impress anyone or a group of persons. It does not matter whether the person is a pastor, pastor's wife, church elder or you all belong to the same choir, youth group or any of the groups in church. It is your personal life. Make the decision and live with the consequences.

Marriageability Traits

Both the potential husband and wife must have compatible personalities. Many experts agree that there are certain traits that make an individual a more suitable partner for making a marriage work. If these elements are present, there is a greater possibility of establishing a successful marriage. These include:

- Similar religious and spiritual interests

- Common beliefs and values

- Emotional stability and no use of drugs

- A willingness to share intimate thoughts and feelings

- Flexibility and Adaptability to situations

- Good communication skills and a conversationalist

- Able to work through problems and resolve conflict

- Respect and appreciation for each other

- The ability to give and receive love

- Comfort in expressing emotions

- Mentally sound and a good sense of humour

Are we compatible?

In addition to the above, marriage was established by God for mankind to share, support and honour one another. These three reasons are fundamental to the success of your marriage. You must consider these reasons carefully and seek someone who is genuinely prepared to share, support and honour you.

All these factors could be considered under the umbrella of compatibility. Many couples ask the question, "Are we compatible?"

Compatibility is about getting along well together with your partner. It describes the harmonious relationship with your partner. The important elements in achieving compatibility include friendship, respect and sexual attraction (not lust). It is important to ensure that these components exist in your relationship.

Is your partner your best friend? Friendship is necessary to keep your relationship going. Do you like your partner? If you don't then there is no need continuing the relationship under the pretext of being in love. If you do not like your partner, do not fake it as you will be exposed with time. You need to spend time to build your friendship. You will need this component as the years go by. Some people claim that they are growing to like the partner. This is significant. Because you can't love someone you do not like nor build intimacy with someone you can not call a friend.

Two important components of compatibility are respect and support. Respecting your partner include considering their feelings, needs and their point of view as well as being faithful in the relationship. Supporting your partner includes establishing confidence in him/her, offering when needed especially in a difficult circumstance.

H. Norman Right explains that the issue of compatibility can mean "how well the intrinsic characteristics of two people fit. Compatibility between individuals can also determine how easily a relationship can be established. However, this provides only the potential for a good marriage; it is necessary, but not sufficient on its own. The more compatible the better, but the potential must be activated and used. No two people are absolutely compatible. It is a matter of becoming compatible during your early years of marriage."

The careful selection of a mate does not guarantee a good marriage. However, it can guarantee you a solid foundation on which to build a workable marriage relationship. It gives you a head start, which is essential in the early years of your marriage.

The words of Kofi Annan, Former Secretary-General of the United Nations, is food for thought and very appropriate to re-iterate here: "To live is to choose. But to choose well, you must know who you are and what you stand for, where you want to go and why you want to get there".

H/C

Words Of Wisdom

"Trust in the lord with your heart

And lean not on your own understanding,

In all your ways acknowledge him,

And he will make your paths straight.

—Proverbs 3:5-6

CHAPTER 4

THE DECISION TIME: TO MARRY OR NOT TO MARRY

Deep Thinking

Now you have selected your mate. This is the time for deep thinking. You do not have to literally close your eyes and just fall in love with the view to getting married. You must do serious personal reflections. It is important to talk to yourself and examine your own motives and needs. It is also very essential to determine your own goals and decide what you want to achieve personally in the relationship. This has nothing to do with your partner. It is about what you want.

What exactly do you want? What do you want in the relationship? Are you simply in love for love sake? Are you in love because it is your hope that the relationship would lead to marriage? This is your life. Think. Your future happiness or sadness would emerge from the result of your deep reflection and analysis. When you have the opportunity to choose between future happiness and future sadness all you need to do is to think. Search for information and advice that will enable you to make a wise decision. Think and think well. When you can't find your way clear, talk to a trusted friend, a family member, a pastor or a counsellor.

Behind the back of your mind should be the word "why". Why did I choose this person? Any justification why I have chosen this person? What are the criteria? Am I making the right decision? Is he/she the right choice for me? What are the special issues that helped to inform my decision? To what extent am I right? What if I have made the wrong decision? Does he/she have all or some of the qualities I want in a future spouse? If not, can I leave with the bad ones?

In all the certainties and uncertainties as to whether you want to get married to your partner or not, scriptures states in Proverbs 3:5-6 that:

Trust in the lord with your heart

And lean not on your own understanding,

In all your ways acknowledged him,

And he will make your paths straight.

What does it mean to trust the Lord with all your heart and lean not on your own understanding? It means that we completely trust God with all that is within us. We simply rely not on anything that we can do on our own strength, and that we give all of the strength we possess, both physically and mentally, to the will of the Holy Spirit. Then God can fulfill his perfect will through us and bring glory to Himself. We do not seek our own gain but desire God to receive all the glory. We get to enjoy what God does for himself.

To lean not on our own understanding means we are not seeking to figure the problem out logically. This is not ours to do. If God is truly the center of our lives, we live for him and him alone. If we really believe that he lives, then we should also believe that we can trust him with all our hearts. The result is the blessing of God falling on the obedient vessel, the vessel that was used to fulfill God's perfect will.

"In all your ways acknowledge him" – this is to fear God in all we do. To fear the Lord is to be wise. We should fear God when we get up in the morning, we should fear God when we start to talk, think, eat, listen, and act. When we are around people we should fear God. This keeps us wise, and most importantly keeps us from sinning (Proverbs 1:7; Exodus 20:20).

Here is the blessing: "He will make your paths straight". Why? Because they are no longer our paths, but His. Since He is perfect, he can't have any fault in Him. So the paths must lead to fulfilling his work, his perfect will, in and through the life he has given.

Mind-set

The decision to get married must fit into your mind-set. You must be ready to accept these mindset changes psychologically. Marriage involves extra responsibilities and commitment and it is not for the faint hearted. It is for the bold, courageous and adventurous people, those who are prepared to move forward. The question is whether you are prepared physically, spiritually, psychologically and financially to move forward.

Are both of you well prepared to get married? This is important. Sometimes, a partner wants to get married because after courting for along time, he/she things the next step is to get married. Without adequate preparation, you would be setting the stage for failure. Sometimes too, when the relationship is deteriorating, the partners feel that the only way to revitalise the relationship is to drift towards marriage. That is also a recipe for failure. For the marriage to work, both of you must want to get married and must also be interested in pursuing it. When one person feels that he or she is being forced into the marriage, that is also a sure sign of failure. Therefore, if both of you are determined to marry, then the sky is your limit; go for it.

Studies proves that, when a man affirms in his decision that he wants to get married, the couple are more probable to be married than if it is the woman who so desires and expresses the concern to tie the knot.

Too Late to Change Your Mind?

It is very normal to have doubts about your relationship. Sometimes our personal expectations are not matched. When you have doubts about your relationship, it does not mean that you have to withdraw from it. It may rather mean that you have to do some homework and talk to your partner about your doubts and fears. It is vital to obtain clarification upon any misgivings and concerns to enable you make up your mind. When you need help, it is important to consult your counsellor to help you to make a decision.

Rev Jeff Vines narrated a story that happened to him, as a young man, on his wedding day, to his congregation at the Christ Church of the Valley, Arizona, USA. Kindly read on; "I was back behind the curtains ready to come out standing with the wedding party waiting on the bride. Robin is at the back with the wedding dress ready to come in and everybody waiting to come in.

I was ready to walk out and got the signal. My father grabbed my arm; I turned and said "Dad, I've got to go."

"No, you don't!" My Dad said. And he gave me the keys to his car and said "you take this key and you go away. Drive out of here and I'm going out there to tell them you changed your mind."

I turned to him and said to my Dad; "Dad, are you crazy? I can't do that!" My Dad said to me, "oh yes you can do that now .But in an hour's time, that opportunity will never arise again."

That was my dad's way of telling me that "when you walk out there, that is it for life!" And then he said; "do you understand that young man?""

After deep soul searching, if you are still unsure about the marriage, you must have the courage to call it off or postpone it. Marriage is not for the fait hearted. Deciding not to marry your partner may be the hardest decision of your life. You must have the courage to stand by your convictions. Such a choice might cause pain and disappointment to some close family and friends, but you would save yourself, and possibly your partner, from an unhappy marriage. Remember that it is your life and you are solely responsible for the decision you make.

H℮/C

FOOD FOR THOUGHT

"Taking a woman is not the problem. Any man can do that. But taking the heart and the thoughts of the woman is the most difficult task."

—An African Proverb

CHAPTER 5

RELEVANT INFORMATION BEFORE THE ALTAR

The following are some of the important information you will need before going to the altar.

Due to the prevalence of various diseases, it has become mandatory in some churches for aspiring couples to go for a medical check-up during their counselling period. The main purpose of this is to ensure that each individual is protected.

• *HIV/AIDS*

HIV stands for Human Immunodeficiency Virus. It attacks the body's immune system - the body's defence against disease - so that it can no longer fight off certain infections and diseases. When someone is diagnosed as having HIV in their body, they are described as being HIV positive.

Most people with HIV are living healthy lives, thanks to the treatment and care available. You can't tell by looking at someone if they are HIV positive. Research proves that about 25 per cent of people don't even know they have the virus. That is why it is so important not to make assumptions and always look after your sexual health and that of your partner.

We think that the result of the medical check-up, will throw light on whether they go ahead and get married. They can still be counselled about the risks and difficulties involved to enable them to make a better judgment. There are couples who are aware of each other's medical problems, who still choose to marry. The important factors are openness and trust.

In London, Nana Kofi, a friend of ours attended a crusade. The guest Pastor invited people who had the HIV/Virus to come forward so he can pray for them. The number of people who voluntarily went forward for prayers was a great shock to him. But more surprising to him was that, a beautiful lady who was sitting next to him also stood up and went forward. He was surprised because he had intended to exchange phone numbers with her and ultimately hoped to date her after their initial acquaintance.

The importance of a medical check-up before marriage cannot be overstated. As already stated, the main purpose of this is to ensure that each individual is protected. For example, it would be extremely unfair for one partner to openly prove their clean bill of health while the other secretly harbours infectious diseases.

• *Sickle Cell*

Many people know a little about sickle cell diseases and therefore may not be aware of the implications to both partners. It is a genetic (inherited) blood disorder in which the red blood cells, which carry oxygen around the body, develop abnormally. Rather than being round and flexible, the sickle red blood cells become shaped like a crescent (or sickle).

Sickle cell disease is a condition that is determined by a single pair of genes (one from each parent). It is acquired from parents and it is not contagious.

Sickle cell Anaemia is not a "black disease." It affects persons of Mediterranean, South Asian, Grecian, Italian, Hispanic, and South America descent.

It is a complex disease. Good quality medical care and living healthily can prevent some serious problems.

If, following the health check, it becomes evident that it would be impossible or grossly inadvisable to marry, then seek counselling and go your separate ways. The counselling will help you to overcome any emotional issues including a sense of guilt or loss. After assessing the available medical evidence, if both partners still want to proceed with the marriage, then that is their choice, as is the decision whether or not to have a family. It is imperative, however, that they are in possession of all available information and know what they are committing themselves to.

Wisdom

Scriptures tells us that "if any man lacks wisdom, let him ask God, who gives to all men generously and without reproach and it will be given to him." James 1:5. You will need to constantly ask the Lord for wisdom in order to sustain your relationship.

You need wisdom in everything you do in the relationship. For example, you need wisdom to communicate with your mate on a daily basis. "My mouth shall speak wisdom; the meditation of my heart shall understand". Psalm 49:3. Scripture also says that we must be quick to listen and slow to speak.

Wisdom, insight or understanding, call it what you will, is needed in conflict management in the relationship. Once you are in a relationship, resolving conflicts with your mate might become an issue. Wisdom is also needed in critical areas such as arguments, handling of would be in-laws and friends and so on.

Wisdom dictates that showing simple courtesies and respect to your mate's friends and family will go a long way to sustain the relationship.

Scripture assures us that even when we are in trouble, we should not think about how to answer the charges, "for I will give you a mouth and wisdom, which none of your adversaries will be able to withstand or contradict". What an assurance. Pray for wisdom and knowledge. Acquire wisdom as insight and experience; do not underestimate its immense value.

The mouth of the righteous utters wisdom, and his tongue speaks justice. Psalm 37:30

Prayer

As Christians, you will need to pray always. If you do not know how to pray, talk to your Pastor. You will need to pray constantly and with commitment. Prayer must be part of your daily life. The Bible says that we are in a spiritual battle against the principalities, against the powers, against the world rulers of this present darkness, against the spiritual hosts of wickedness in the heavenly places. The devil is vigilant to this battle and very subtle. Satan disguises himself as a prince of light and can enter your relationship when you least expect. You must therefore pray without ceasing.

Some superficial developments in your relationship might appear trivial and may be easily solved. At other times, they might not be what you initially thought. The problems could be more serious than you imagined. Fervent prayer with an unshakable faith will help you.

You must pray daily for yourselves, the unity, peace and happiness, as well as the sustenance of your relationship. Above all, pray for God's presence and love in your relationship. The most powerful tool you have as a would be couple is to pray together: the power of two. There is a potent unifying effect when you join together and lift up prayers to the Lord. The Bible states that "for where two or three are gathered in my name, there I am in the midst of them. Matthew 18: 20.

Don't forget to pray for your mate or would be spouse. You know your would be spouse's desires, wants, needs and goals. Lift these needs in prayer before the Lord daily. Ask for wisdom and knowledge to enable him/her to make better judgements in his/her daily life. Pray to the Lord for strength and good health for your would be spouse.

God is the creator of marriage as an institution. He is in fact the manufacturer of marriage and therefore knows the product better than anyone else.

No one actually knows a product better than the manufacturer. My wife and I bought a Honda CRV automatic vehicle. It was just five years old. We noticed that there was noise at the back of the vehicle. I advised that we take the vehicle to a garage just around the corner, not far away from our house. The mechanic checked everything and worked on the vehicle, yet the problem persisted. The second mechanic misdiagnosed it while the third suspected the break system. He tinkered with it for two days and still the noise was there. He actually worsened the situation by creating another problem on the vehicle.

It was now time for the annual MOT and so my wife suggested that we send it to the Honda garage in Loughton, Essex. UK. I agreed. At the Honda reception, we complained about the issue. Immediately, the

Manager said, "there is a shortage of oil at the back of the vehicle. We will put in some oil and the problem will stop". True to his word, when the vehicle came out from the garage, the noise had stopped. It drove perfectly well like a brand new car. We abandoned our plans to sell it off at a cheaper price and we used it for several years. God has the solutions to your relationship problems and challenges. Go to Him for the solutions and surely He will provide them.

Words of Wisdom

"What makes life interesting, what makes a conversation stimulating is people with differing points of view. Those who need others to think and act exactly the way they do are often masking insecurities, and have a deep-seated need to have their views and actions confirmed in the behaviour and thought of others. Disagreements happen in any relationship where more than one person is involved; it's inevitable"

—T.D Jakes

CHAPTER 6

COURTSHIP: A STEP TOWARDS THE ALTAR

Importance

After dating for a while, it is likely that the relationship will move to a new stage. The man invariably initiates the move, often encouraged by the woman's behaviour, and he makes his intentions known to the woman. The emphasis is on intention; a verbalised intention to share the future together as husband and wife.

However, relationships do not progress to formal courtship in every case. Sometimes, there is some indication that the relationship may not work in the long term and one or other partner may stall for time in order to be absolutely sure of making the right decision.

The courtship period is a time of close interaction. This builds confidence, understanding, trust and reassurance. This is the time when both parties must make an effort to learn more detailed information about each other. For example, you must be confident that you have taken the time to get to know about and understand your partner's background and circumstances. As a matter of priority, you need to know your partner inside out, their public and their private self. Blinded by "love", several individuals accept their partners as they are. They tend, mistakenly, to think that certain questions are taboo, might cause offence or can always be asked later.

This period is also about moulding each other's character. You become responsible for, and to, each other. You must look out for certain habits or patterns of behaviour. Those who are irresponsible before marriage, tend to be irresponsible during marriage. If you are unable to persuade your partner to change during the courtship, there is a little chance of succeeding after marriage. For example, if you are aware your partner is an alcoholic, a drug user, or abusive and violent, but you fail to persuade him or her to change, then you need to think seriously before committing to a shared lifetime under these conditions. At this point, there is no obligation to marry your partner with a view to changing him or her. If you marry your partner out of sympathy, or believing that things will improve once you are married, you are likely to create serious problems for yourself in the future. The likelihood is that you will either have to adapt to the person's behaviour or call it a day.

Overlooked Differences

Most differences tend to be overlooked while the couple is dating and courting. There are some who believe that they are made or created for each other. Hence, when there are basic differences between them, these are denied, ignored or deemed acceptable. According to the saying, 'opposites attract'. When these differences are overlooked, it is highly likely they will become the basis for future arguments or criticism in the marriage. Unresolved differences can result in a fragile relationship and weaken the very foundation of the relationship. Watch out for the "small prints".

At this level of commitment, conversations should become more open, taking place between the couple, in confidence. Communication must be honest and intimate and trust becomes very important and contributes to strengthening the relationship. This is possibly the time to tell your partner certain secrets. Remember that if your partner is not able to forgive you, there is no way you will be forgiven after you are married. The manner in which you approach any difficult issues is crucial.

Essential Questions

In summary, communication during courtship should be open. Confidentiality, commitment and trust are vital if the relationship is to be built on strong foundations.

Some issues to consider should include:

A partner's former relationships: Be reasonable and non-judgemental. This is a sensitive issue. People sometimes behave differently under different circumstances. Some may want to hide past relationships by being less than honest. The fear of being viewed as too promiscuous or 'cheap', prevents one from telling the truth. However, it is better to tell the truth now than to let your partner hear from other sources.

Ask if there were any children from the previous relationship. If there are, can you deal with that comfortably? Remember that these children will be part of your relationship for the rest of your life. Office romances sometimes figure in people's relationships, especially when an ex happens to work in the same organisation or is close by. Find out as much information as possible by asking questions about the extent of the relationship and make absolutely certain it has completely ended. Do not leave any issue to chance, otherwise you may find yourself competing against shadows.

It is important to find out about a partner's health status. In this age of HIV/AIDs and other sexually transmitted diseases, it is essential to find out whether your partner has been screened for HIV as well as other Sexually Transmitted Diseases. Finding out about such serious illnesses has nothing to do with trust. Please do not be foolish when your life could be at risk. Your life is of paramount importance and you would be wise to remember that dead men don't count. In addition, confirm the sickle cell status is clear, as well as other medical conditions.

Sometimes probing too deeply may make your partner uncomfortable, but remember; you are not asking them anything you would not willingly reveal about yourself and any reluctance to give you such information may tell you all you need to know. You may choose to find other ways of obtaining the necessary information, but you must ask yourself how beneficial the information will be, what will you do with such information and will it influence your decision about the future of your relationship?

On the other hand, if you are fortunate enough to be the first person your partner has been involved with, then you will have other issues to address.

Find out about their current job. Do they have plans for the future and, if so, what measures have they put in place to ensure these plans are realised? Is your partner satisfied with their current position? Is he or she ambitious and interested in climbing the career ladder? If so, do they have a realistic and achievable strategy in place?

What are your partner's expectations in your future marriage? Are they too high or low? What are the anticipated roles of a wife or husband in the future home? What is your partner's understanding of companionship, cooperation and love within a marriage partnership? What is your partner's view on raising a family?

Are there any secrets in the family that you should know of? Have your partner's parents given their lives to Christ? Do any family members belong to a cult or secret society? What has been their Christian background in general? Insist politely on details. If you are confused by any information or responses you are given, and become unsure, talk to your counsellor or Pastor as soon as possible.

What is your partner's understanding of respect? What does it really mean to him/her? Find out what he/she likes or dislikes and what causes them to be frustrated or anxious in life.

Making the Proposal

A formal proposal is made regarding your intention and a positive response is received from the woman before courtship formally begins. The process differs within each culture and tradition. However in most cultures, it is the man who proposes. This has some mystery surrounding it and we believe it should be left that way. Men by nature are hunters and they in most cases respect what they have struggled to achieve, the fruit of their labour. It is perfectly acceptable for the woman to apply subtle pressure, especially if the man seems to be indecisive. If the man is playing games or suffers from commitment phobia, do not waste your time. This also applies equally to the man. If the woman is wasting your time with all sorts of excuses, please do not allow yourself to be used and then cast aside.

Sometimes, people play a waiting game with the view to bidding for time. Men for example, delay making a decision to be sure the lady they have in mind will agree to their proposal. Women also play similar games, perhaps waiting for the right man to propose at the right time.

Family Involvement

Prior to making a formal proposal, discuss it with your family. This is important in order to show respect and to honour your parents and family members, as they deserve. The scripture commands us to honour our father and mother so that our days may be long. The blessing of the family is important for your future happiness on this journey.

It is a fact that whenever a new relationship begins, each partner brings a multitude of family and friends into the equation. We all have family members whose opinion we respect and who have our best interest at heart. These are the core members you need to speak with prior to making any formal introduction, making or accepting a proposal.

Your family may have high expectations of you due to your education, religious upbringing, background, social standing and other intangibles. Therefore, when you present your prince charming or beautiful princess and it does not meet their expectation, it becomes a bitter pill to swallow. Mothers especially always pray that their children will bring home the best mate that will meet their expectations. For that reason, they are always on the lookout. If your choice does not meet their set standard, you may be in for a faulty start in your relationship.

However, we are in a real world. Your future in-laws are prone to change their mind when they realise with time that you are more than what they thought about you. It means that you must be able to justify yourself worthy of being an in-law. They will watch you closely; do their own intelligence gathering to ensure that they are welcoming a prince or princess to their home.

It is not easy for parents to accept a new member into their family, sometimes it's simply for security reasons. No parents would welcome an in-law who may, for example, expose their vulnerabilities and family secrets. Therefore, you would be welcome with an open arms but with caution. With time, when you grow to understand the family politics and beliefs, you would be able to adjust yourself.

Friends

Friends also play a very vital role in your lives. When growing up, especially during the teenage years, the network of friendship you build help to shape your ideas and provides you with a sense of belonging and support as well as exchange of information and ideas. You are able to receive security, information as well as share problems, provide and receive advice. Therefore, it is imperative that you involve friends in terms of consultation, reasoning together and decision making. This is important because your friends may or may not like your choice and that may influence your final decision. Therefore, the essential thing to do is to find out from your intimate friends what they think about your choice. But at the end of the day, the choice is yours and you must be able to stand by your decision you have made.

The Pastors Advice

You will need information and advice from your Pastor. If you are already courting, inform your Pastor as a matter of courtesy. He may be in a position to provide helpful facts, advice and guidance that could possibly save you from unnecessary disappointment. He is experienced in providing the necessary spiritual assistance to guide you and you disregard this information at your peril. You require God's blessing in this matter.

It is important that you begin attending counselling sessions in your church. If there are no marriage counsellors in your church, make enquiries about a good local Christian marriage counsellor and seek advice. It is in your own interests and, for your partner's too, that you follow this course of action.

Piece of Advice

An important piece of advice is to devote some special time to the relationship, allowing it to develop, before announcing it to the world. You need to establish a firm foundation, otherwise, your courtship stands the risk of being blown away by the wind. A new relationship is much more fragile and susceptible to small cracks and these need attending to, in order to avoid the relationship crumbling prematurely.

WORDS OF WISDOM

"By wisdom a house is built, and through under-standing it is established. Through Knowledge its rooms are filled with rare and beautiful treasures."

—(Proverbs 24; 3-4)

CHAPTER 7

Premarital counselling: Gaining knowledge and information

Ignorance

The average man or woman is likely to spend several weeks and months reading books about how to pass a driving test. Once you pass, you will be issued with your legal driving licence entitling you to drive for a lifetime. This also means that you have to abide by the rules otherwise, you risk losing your licence.

Yet, that same average man will meet a woman (or vice versa) and move into marriage without the slightest idea of what he or she is getting into. The sad thing is that they believe, rightly or wrongly, that they are in love and therefore have taken a bold step. Unfortunately, getting married has nothing to do with being a bold man or courageous woman. Otherwise the bold and courageous would never divorce. It is a totally different ball game. Therefore, like driving, you need an instructor. There are many very good and highly experienced ones to offer you guidance.

My wife Dorothy had a very experienced driving instructor. She spent several weeks practising, and passed the first time. On the other hand, I decided not to take an instructor and relied on my own skills, experience and ideas about driving. In addition, I read several books and watched DVDs and videos. I also read and watched relevant links on the Internet. It did not work for me the first or second time. In the end, it cost me more time and resources, as well as the investment in a skilled instructor.

Several couples spend more time and resources on planning for their weddings. To them, the half a day ceremony is the most important day of their lives. No thought is giving to marriage counselling. The irony is that parents, Church members and well-wishers participate fully in the wedding. They put on their best clothes and are very pleased to remain as spectators on the 'big' day. They sing, dance, bring gifts and cards and take pictures, as well as taking an active part in the reception.

If the Church does not insist on it as a pre-requisite to the wedding, then couples often marry in ignorance. Even in the Church, premarital counselling is left to the Pastors who are very busy with other schedules within and outside the Church.

In the Bible, the closest we come to premarital counselling is St Paul's advice in 1 Corinthians 7. He encourages people to remain single, but states that they should marry if they cannot exercise self-control. For, as he says, it is better to marry than to be aflame with passion. He warns that marriage will bring challenges and pressures, and adds that it is difficult for married people to serve the Lord whole heartedly, because part of their focus will be on pleasing each other. We also read what an ideal marriage should be, which roles the husband and wife should fulfil and how they should behave as parents. This is highlighted in the New Testament, specifically in Corinthians, Ephesians and Peter. However, there are no clear Biblical examples or specific instructions for premarital guidance.

What is Premarital Counselling?

Premarital counselling is largely education, advice and information-giving about marriage. It enlightens couples and shows them the realities of married life. It enables them to deliberate on issues, which can affect their relationship. It also provides certain preparatory training including communication skills; conflict and relationship management _ that can cause divorce or create serious problems in the relationship or future marriage.

In premarital counselling, there is a body of knowledge which those being counselled need to know. The Counsellor is more than a teacher. The Counsellor's task is to help the couple make discoveries: about what the Bible teaches on marriage, about themselves and about their future partner and about what can weaken or strengthen their marriage. It encourages attitudes and behavioural change. Rational skills are taught and opportunities are given to put them into practice.

It might involve problem solving or crisis counselling since any courtship or marriage relationship will encounter problems and even crises. At times it will be necessary to refer a couple to a specialised Counsellor, better qualified to handle a particular problem or desperate situation. Premarital counselling is partnership counselling with the Holy Spirit being the Master Counsellor. The Holy Spirit can give the Counsellor insights and wisdom beyond his or her own understanding.

Premarital counselling also involves the Counsellor developing an ongoing relationship with the couple, offering them another avenue in problem solving as they enter marriage. It is the duty of the Counsellor to pray for the couple regularly. In premarital counselling, the Counsellor's key verse is James1:19 ("...be quick to listen and slow to speak..."). The Premarital Counsellor will do as much listening as talking. He will encourage the couple to talk about themselves to each other and to discover for themselves the truth from God's word. The Counsellor should not lecture during the counselling session. Premarital counselling is intended to gently guide the couple to openly share information with each other and with their Counsellor. As with all counselling, the content of pre-marriage guidance is strictly confidential.

(Adapted from A Pre-marriage Counselling Handbook by Alan and Donna Goerz.)

Reasons for Premarital Guidance

Many marriages today are like the proverbial house built upon sand. They have been built on a very weak foundation. This is not surprising. The evidence is at news stands everywhere. Headlines about well-known personalities, so called celebrities, and TV presenters, actors and actresses, popular musicians and sometimes Pastors, and others who are divorcing or cheating on their mates, fill the front pages of the tabloids and magazines.

When we read romantic books, magazines and watch romantic films and television programmes, we are given a distorted picture of marriage. This misleading and unhelpful view, showing popular misconceptions of marriage, is a recipe for disaster. It leads to unrealistic expectations and problems. Most people receive their information by observing their parents, brothers, sisters, aunties and uncles and other adults in their immediate circle. They accept, often without question, that what they see or observe is the correct information they need before embarking upon their own marriage.

A prospective bride and groom may come together for the wrong reasons, to escape from a difficult home situation, for example, or to add excitement to their lives, perhaps even to conceal an accidental pregnancy. Other misguided reasons include marrying to escape from loneliness, getting married to be like one's peers. Sometimes, the reasons and motives for marriage are not strong enough to withstand the challenges and storms of daily life.

Though it is an established fact that premarital counselling is effective, it has been proven that especially in these days, it is necessary and beneficial to married couples. Talking to some happily married Christian couples we have personally counselled, as well as to those who have had the benefit of counselling elsewhere, we are able to agree that it has contributed to the success of their marriages. We have not received any petitions for divorce nor settled any. We pray that those who benefited from counselling will be a shining example to others.

Premarital counselling is about establishing proper foundations for a strong and healthy marriage. It is preventive counselling, offering immunisation against possible problems, which act like harmful infections, within marriage.

It is concerned with creating a union that can survive the pressures of an uncertain future. It seeks to prevent and pre-empt marriage problems and personal conflicts that could contribute to making the future unfulfilled and miserable. Most people, including Christians, assume that certain problems and challenges happen to others but not to them. They tend to think that they are resistant to problems and therefore will not go for premarital counselling.

There is also the tendency for some people to believe that because they are Christians, problems and challenges faced by other people will not affect them. Consequently, they think that it is not necessary to seek premarital counselling. They would only do so if it is a pre-condition of their marriage being approved by the church.

There are some partners who attend the premarital counselling simply so that they are given the chance to marry in their church. This is because with some of the churches, the policy is that without attending premarital counselling, you cannot have your wedding in the church premises and thus your marriage will not be approved by the church.

This type of partner attends the sessions with a certain attitude. Some even consider it an intrusion into their personal life and behave defensively as if they are merely tolerating the counsellor until the session ends. Such people do not participate fully and will only reluctantly answer certain questions when pressed for answers.

Goals of Premarital Counselling

1. To help the couple learn about God's plan for marriage.

2. To lead each partner to Christ and on towards spiritual maturity.

3. To help each partner learn to know himself or herself better.

4. To help the couple know each other better

5. To help the couples clarify whether they are the right partners for each other and whether the time is right for marriage

6. To help the couple find freedom from the possible cycle of their family's marriage failures.

7. To help the couple build a sense of adventure towards marriage. "With God in this relationship, the potential for success is excellent."

8. To help the couple learn communication skills through teaching, by example and through role-playing.

9. To help the couple discover areas of potential problems and learn skills for managing problems in marriage.

10. To help the couple develop a new way of relating to their extended families.

11. To help the couple develop a plan for managing finances in their home.

12. To help the couple overcome misconceptions about sex and understand God's plan for sex within marriage.

13. To help the couple prepare for the wedding.

Adapted from Pre-Marriage Counselling Handbook by Alan & Donna Goerz. A Pre-Marriage Counselling Handbook, Challenge and Family Ministries.

Commencement of Premarital Counselling

There are people who can court for so long that the relationship runs out of steam. Marriage is for those who are spiritually, physically, socially and psychologically mature. Therefore, when the couple is quite certain that they want to get married, they must then see their Pastor and arrange for premarital counselling. While we would not recommend that you take a lifelong decision in haste, we would equally not recommend that you court for several years. We would recommend a minimum period of one year and a maximum courtship of three years.

Premarital counselling should begin before public announcements have been made or dates have been set for the customary or traditional marriage or church wedding. Premarital counselling is intended primarily to help the couples shed more light on whether they are the right partners for each other. It will also enable them to determine whether it is the right time to marry.

With some churches, there is a waiting period within which the counselling begins, after the pastors have been informed. Within this period, a couple may decide they are not meant for each other Counsellors cannot play God by saying with absolute certainty that a couple's relationship will or will not succeed and therefore, at this point, they must accept the couple's decision. However, sometimes there are indications that it might not work. The counselling can slow couples down so they can spend more time in serious thought and reflection before making a final decision. They may also decide that they need to wait a while longer before getting married. Sometimes after premarital counselling, they may decide that they are not meant for each other and may therefore end plans to marry.

H∘C

WORDS OF WISDOM

If any of you lacks wisdom, let him ask God, who gives to all men generously and without reproaching, and it will be given him. But let him ask in faith, with no doubting, for he who doubts is like a wave of the sea that is driven and tossed by the wind. For that person must not suppose that a double-minded man, unstable in all his ways, will receive anything from the Lord.
—(James 1: 5-8)

CHAPTER 8

ENGAGEMENT & TRADITIONAL MARRIAGE

Engagement

Engagement is an assurance or a promise, normally from a man to a woman to marry her. It is also referred to as the betrothal. It is the most important step leading to marriage and is the usual precursory action or vocalisation indicating an intent to marry.

There are established ways in every culture about how engagement is done. In the western world, engagement is not a serious thing. A man will court a woman for some time. After a while, the man wishes to move the relationship a step further by proposing to the woman. Normally the man asks the question "Will you marry me?" while kneeling, sitting or standing. Between the two people and without any witnesses, the man then puts a ring on the woman's finger. In this way, the formal traditional marital process has begun.

From an African perspective, depending on the tribe, tradition and culture, steps are taken to inform the woman's family of the man's intention to marry their daughter. A suitable date is then agreed upon for the ceremony to take place. It is important to note that it is not an individual's affair but that of the parents, family and sometimes the community.

The Role of the Family

The decision to marry may be personal, but it necessarily invites the active involvement of the whole family. The extent of the family's involvement would largely depend on how close individuals are to family members. Therefore, if both partners are close to their families, the importance cannot be overlooked. Families are more relevant, and should be involved, if they are very influential in the lives of you and your parents. The input of the family regarding who you are marrying carries a great deal of weight.

Scripture advises children to obey their parents in the Lord for this is right and states in the First Commandment, that children should honour their father and mother, with a promise, so 'that it may be well with you and you may live long in the land that the Lord has given you". (Exodus 20:12)

It is unwise to rebel against your parents. Sometimes, there may be criticism from your parents or family about the choice of a partner. This requires discussion and compromise, not silent hostility.

It is not advisable to disregard your parents' advice, eloping and marrying your partner in secret. You will not receive their blessings that you need to carry into the marriage. If you defy your parents and run away with your partner, the sad but inevitable effect is that, in time, the "romantic love" you enjoy will fade and as the emotions stabilise, life will return to normal and then problems will invariably begin. This will show itself in all aspects of your married life. Unfortunately, marriage is not a child's game. It is for the mature. You need to be both psychologically and physically mature.

Once you have decided to marry, some family members may be very active and play a central role in the activities. They may have the time and experience to organise proceedings. They do this out of love and as part of the public relations process to enable the family's name to be held in high esteem.

This role, however, will reduce after the ceremony. It is important to note that you are part of an extended family. Relatives will not go away simply because you think some of them are a nuisance. This is always going to be a possibility. You simply cannot throw away your family and adopt someone else's family as your own.

As you grow up, you need to be mature, sensible and responsible. All issues concerning the families must be approached with some sensitivity. Respect is the key word here. If you give respect to your partner's family, you will earn their respect in return. Compromises will have to be made in order to sustain and nurture the relationship. One of the secrets to a successful marriage is to develop good relations with your spouse's family. In some cultures, close family members, such as the mother, father, uncles and aunties are revered and hold a great deal of influence.

The Relevance of the Engagement/Traditional Marriage

In Africa, engagement is a big ceremony. The wedding is seen as a "Christian" celebration. Depending on which country, culture or tradition you come from, the engagement is highly important and very significant to both the parents and families. There is some argument as to whether the engagement ceremony is a full marriage. The ceremony formally brings the two families together. The covenant set between them is agreed on by the witnesses present.

Western cultures do not have such an elaborate traditional ceremony. Therefore, most writers of marriage issues are silent on the importance and significance of the engagement. Interestingly, Some African writers follow this way of thinking.

To the Western writers, the wedding ceremony is the recognised formalisation of marriage. However, to most Africans, the traditional marriage is the real marriage covenant. Some African Pastors are confused when confronted with this issue. The importance of the traditional marriage cannot be over emphasised. This ceremony establishes a bond between the couple, where their families pronounce their blessings. In most cases, there are men of God present, who also bless the marriage. This act confirms it as a full marriage. The woman joins the husband in his house and the marriage relationship then starts. There is full sexual consummation.

The two families are bonded together and are accepted into each other's family. Family members travel from various parts of the country to witness and celebrate the marriage ceremony.

In this type of marriage, the man or woman cannot seek divorce on a whim or superficial excuse because of the involvement of the two families. Generally, the marriages are intended for life, as the families will not entertain even the slightest hint of divorce. They will tell both partners that marriage is for life and that divorce is not the answer. Whatever problems the couple may have, the families will be interested in sitting down and listening to the two sides before offering advice and making a judgement.

We had the opportunity of participating in solving marriage problems of this kind both in Ghana and abroad. In all these cases, the families agreed that they should go for counselling. By the grace of God, these couples are still married, three to five years after the issue. We have not forgotten one particular case in which an elder concluded, "We have heard both parties. Let them go and work out their differences, seek help and we shall meet in a year's time to evaluate the progress and take a decision". They are still married. Since it is not easy to divorce under the traditional marriage system, couples are more focused on finding ways to work out the relationship than finding a way of escape.

The "white" wedding is the crowning glory of the marriage process for us as Christians.

H/C

WORDS OF WISDOM

"Where there is no guidance, a people falls; but in an abundance of counselors there is safety."

—Proverbs 11;14

CHAPTER 9

THE WEDDING CEREMONY: THE MARRIAGE BEGINS

The "D – Day"

We all heard the words clearly at the church on our wedding day. "William, will you have this woman as your wedded wife, to live together after God's ordinance in the holy estate of matrimony? Will you love her, comfort her, and keep her in sickness and in health; and forsaking all others, keep thee only unto her, so long as both of you shall live?"

I answered, "Yes, I will".

Then the Priest turned to Dorothy.

"Will you have this man as your wedded husband, to live together after God's ordinance in the holy estate of Matrimony? Will you obey him, and serve him, love, honour and keep him in sickness and in health, and forsaking all others, keep thee only unto him, so long as ye both shall live?"

She answered, "Yes, I will".

Then there was a loud shout of Hallelujah, Praise the Lord! Followed by a loud clap from the invited guests and church members.

"By the authority vested in me, I pronounce you man and wife. God be your helper". And the best part – "you may kiss your bride." The priest concluded.

Suddenly, everything changed about us; a mystery that was inexplicable to us. The spiritual significance of the wedding cannot be over emphasised. Our world changed. Suddenly, we found ourselves with each other. There is something mysterious about marriage that seems beyond explanation to the newly married couple. Marriage looks spiritual and it is. You suddenly find yourself in a sacred time-honoured institution. There is an inner glow within. You look different. You feel different. You look and feel satisfied and fulfilled, confident and hopeful for the future.

After our wedding, our good friend and best man, Sony Fynn-Williams of blessed memory, sent us the following joke; the story is entitled; *the guilty are always afraid.* Kindly read on;

The bride and the groom arrived at the Church and the wedding   ceremony began.

Pastor: "If there is anybody here that does not want this couple to be joined together in holy matrimony, he or she should speak out now."

A man from the extreme end of the church stood up and walked towards the altar. As the bride saw the man coming closer, she fainted. The bridegroom and the whole congregation were in confusion.

When the man got to the front, the pastor asked, "Why don't you want these people to be joined together?"

Man: "I could not hear your voice clearly from the back, Sir, so I decided to come and tell you that the speaker is faulty!!"

The Counsellor's Role

The Counsellor is a change specialist. His or her job is to help deal with the changes that come into your lives and to facilitate changes that will improve your lives. He/she understands the change process taking place in your life.

The Counsellor will provide you with various information about what to expect on the wedding day. He or she will also explain to you the sacredness of the vows you will be making on the wedding day. It is important that you discuss your fears and expectations with the Counsellor. He or she is there to provide you with information, advice and to answer all your questions in confidence.

If the Counsellor is a member of your church, he or she will inform the Pastor about your progress. As a result, the Church will permit you to have your wedding because you have done as the church policy requires regarding marriage.

The Family

The family is instrumental in shaping who we are. The very least you can do to honour them is to allow them to be involved in planning the wedding. Even if you consider that by virtue of your wealth or status, their involvement is not necessary, involve them in a very subtle way. Respect your family members. You can't do this on your own. Talk to them about the wedding. They may have some vital information to give you or some helpful advice to offer. It is your choice, but your parents and siblings may want to see themselves as part of the organisation. Do give them progress reports from time to time.

Weddings should always be joyous occasions. The decision to have a wedding will spread, to your surprise, by word of mouth. Distant relations, as well as members of the family whom you have never seen before, will suddenly appear. There will be those with strong views on how to organise the occasion. You might not want their views, but for the sake of family unity, you will need extra patience to accommodate them. Organising a wedding event brings with it stress, anger and misunderstanding. However, your ability to deal with all these aspects will help you to become a well-fulfilled and more mature person. You will gain their respect. You may never have the opportunity again, in a lifetime, to make such an impression.

In the barrage of counselling and advice, there will be wisdom. It will be helpful to have the many different shades of family opinion but, in the end, the decision is yours. This is the greatest time in your life to perform your public relations. Make sure you involve your family members when preparing your final invitation list. Unfortunately, or perhaps fortunately, you are not alone. You were born into a family and therefore need to approach issues concerning the family with the sensitivity and respect it deserves.

Network of Friends

Your relationship with each other's friends also has an impact on your marriage. If you see eye to eye with your spouse's friends, you broaden your network of friendship. This is a big secret you must never forget. These friends can make or break your marriage in future. The reality is that we all have very good friends whose opinions we respect and sometimes we tend to listen to them more than we do to our parents. These friends can exert a positive or negative influence on us. When it comes to an important occasion like a wedding, we will definitely listen to their views. The friends you have can be a good source for organisation. That is what friends are for. In time of joy and the need for help, you call on them. Inform your friends about your wedding and find out from them how they can help you with ideas, resources and time.

Event Management/Budget

If you have the means to hire an Event Manager to manage the wedding, then that may prove a useful option. That is your choice. Be careful to tell the manager what you want. Discuss with him/her what your budget is and detail your plans. Do this with as many Event Managers as possible. You must know what you want, otherwise you may expose yourself to unnecessary and expensive products, exceeding your budget and not having the wedding you hoped for.

Weddings are very big business. It can be a very expensive undertaking. We have attended several wedding shows and ceremonies in London and Milton Keynes in the UK. We have been involved in the management of several weddings and can only conclude that it can be very expensive depending on your taste.

We calculated that if you want to have a white wedding, then it is important that you plan ahead and save some money for the occasion. Better planning results in better outcomes. You don't have to depend on projected help and you won't have to anticipate the size of the budget your extended family will provide for you to plan around. "A bird in the hand is worth more than ten in the bush", so goes the adage. You need to plan with the money available so that if you receive extra from other sources, it will be a bonus. You may decide to use it towards the organisation.

It is important to cut costs. Sew your dress according to the size of your material. Organise your wedding according to how full your pocket is. Many individuals borrow from a variety of sources to finance their wedding, including from parents, banks, friends, loan sharks, credit unions and through the use of credit cards. It is crucial to plan ahead.

Where one of the partners is richer than the other, this should be counted as a blessing. Sometimes, depending on the culture, most often it is the man who pays a greater percentage of the bills. The woman may be extremely rich and might decide to undertake a bigger portion of the bills. This should be done with the view that the love that binds you transcends the money being used for the wedding ceremony. It should be seen as an act of giving and sharing, to begin a fruitful relationship. Sometimes, parents decide to foot the bill or make a contribution towards it. You must thank God and the parents for their help.

Whatever your situation, it is not advisable to overspend to the extent that you start your married life with a huge debt. This will mean that you will start life with the main aim being paying off the debt. This can cause tension in your marriage. You will need to enjoy the early years of marriage unencumbered with such problems. Quality time should be spent enjoying and planning for the future and adjusting to your newly established relationship and home instead of thinking about how to pay debts.

The Wedding Day

Congratulations! This is a brand new day. People will come to celebrate with you. It is a very big step unto the unknown and a very public statement of commitment. After all, it is about the celebration of your marriage. You may spend several months and sleepless nights working hard to make the day a perfect one. Sometimes things might go wrong. There might be delays with the planned activities, such as the church, catering, or music. But the secret for the success of the day is to smile. Smile when difficult situations are brought to your attention. Never allow anything to spoil the day. It will never happen again. To smile throughout is the secret to the success of the day.

Pray and ask for God's guidance before you enter the church. Moreover, pray also during the ceremony as well as the reception.

Invited Guests

People love weddings. There are some people who will attend a wedding uninvited. Similarly, there are those who will hear of the wedding through a friend or the grapevine and will want to surprise you. You may be surprised, therefore, that you invited 100 people and 200 turn up. Count it all as an unexpected joy that you have people to celebrate with you on such an important occasion.

On the other hand, there are some people who will be disappointed to find out that many of the invited guests did not attend. When this happens, just put on a smile and do not allow it to ruin your day. They may have valid reasons, and if not, the people who matter will be present.

Your human relations also count. How popular you are in a church, community or among your peers, as well as the influence of your parents may also determine the crowd.

My wife and I are involved in Event Management, specifically weddings and so have some knowledge and expertise in this area. When planning the reception, we would inform the prospective couple about their anticipated guests. They might then cut down on the figures in order to cut cost. Sometimes we ask them how many people they would like to invite, and for example, some would suggest 100, "because we don't know many people". We would then advise them to double the number or add an extra fifty. Our experience shows us that depending on how big your church is, the family you come from, your circle of friends, work place and so forth, these would determine the estimated number of guests to expect.

Invited guests will usually bring gifts, cards and enjoy the food and drinks as well as the programmed entertainment at the reception. Don't be anxious if you think you don't know how to dance. You can always work on something with your friends and immediate family members. Just enjoy the day. Keep telling yourselves that this is the day that the Lord has made and we will rejoice in it.

The Honeymoon: After the Wedding

After the wedding is your greatest moment. Both partners always anticipate an exciting honeymoon. Some honeymoons are perfect, but in whatever situation you may find yourself, please do not forget that it is just the beginning of the marriage.

The stresses and strains of the wedding will take their toll. You will need to relax. However, there are those who will have extra energy and adrenalin who will want to make a symbolic use of the night. This is completely normal and acceptable. The couple may want to enjoy sex because there will be no feelings of guilt and being married will add to the excitement and intimacy of a really special encounter as they embark on their marriage. For those who will be having their first sexual experience, sex may be very different from what you have been told or read. You will be having a real, highly personal and totally unique experience.

Surprises and Disappointments

There will be disappointments. For the Christian man who has saved himself with a view to meeting a virgin, he may experience the greatest shock of his life. When a man is not told the truth about past relationships, it leads to disappointments with serious repercussions on a marriage. A Christian brother who had saved himself since infancy, experienced a shocking discovery when during his honeymoon, he found that his newly wedded wife had been unexpectedly and disappointingly promiscuous. Unfortunately, he could not take any action because he had not asked questions about the lady's past relationships. He admitted making a mistake. But that is life. He had to learn to accept the wife as she was, and to seek further counselling on the issue.

In another case, a lady found out to her amazement that the man she married was not circumcised. To her, this was against her tradition and beliefs. The men from her tribe are circumcised at an early age. All her life, she had only ever seen circumcised men. Regrettably, she had failed to ask any intimate questions during the courtship period. She was too much in love and therefore took things for granted. She assumed that her then fiancée was circumcised.

If you have never discussed the issue of sex, this is the best time for you to do so in an open manner. There is no need to be shy and bury your head in the sand or avert your eyes from it. If you do not take the opportunity when it presents itself, you may regret it later. Talk about every issue you want to know. Seek clarification and explanations. Talk about what makes you tick, your likes and dislikes. There is no way your partner will be able to know what you like. There are people who think that talking about sex makes you "dirty". This is a very important and enjoyable shared activity; an important part of a marriage and hopefully, you will be doing it for the rest of your life. Therefore, the more you pay attention and have constructive fruitful discussions with your spouse about it, the better you will enjoy your marriage. Let the few passionate moments you share in a day be worth it. Never opt for a boring sex life.

And there are further surprises. There is always the fear that you may not match up to your spouse's expectations. For the first time, a lady might be worried as to what her husband will think about her nudity. For example, if the lady is used to using too many artificial accessories to enhance her beauty, she may have to remove most of these artificial items. The honeymoon period brings you face to face with each other. Now you have each other for 24 hours. You have to make use of the time as you want and deem fit.

Everything of a personal nature will be revealed once the marriage progresses. Issues that have been swept under the carpet will surface and secrets will rear their ugly heads. Every concern will need to be dealt with and communications between you will have to be excellent, from the onset, to enable you to enjoy your marriage.

H⸰C

WORDS OF WISDOM

"Let your heart hold fast my words;
keep my commandments, and live;
do not forget, and do not turn away from
the words of my mouth.
Get wisdom; get insight.
Do not forsake her, and she will keep you;
love her, and she will guard you.
The beginning of wisdom is this: Get wisdom,
and whatever you get, get insight.
Prize her highly, and she will exalt you;
she will honor you if you embrace her.
She will place on your head a fair garland;
she will bestow on you a beautiful crown."

—(Proverbs 4: 4-9)

CHAPTER 10

RELEVANT INFORMATION FOR A BETTER FOUNDATION

The Difference Between A Man And A Woman.

How interesting. Two people: unique individuals with different personalities and experiences, from different backgrounds, tribes, nationalities, environment, meet each other and agree to marry. Each person brings his or her own perspective, including history, into the marriage. According to the Bible, when God performed the first marriage ceremony between Adam and Eve in the Garden of Eden, He charged them to be fruitful, to multiply, to replenish the earth and to subdue it. Since then, instead of this command being followed, men and women often use their differences to stay divided and uncooperative.

Scriptures

The scripture tells us that God created man and woman. Genesis 5:2 states that "He created them male and female." Some Men of God and Christian counsellors believe that the genesis of all the marital problems emanates from the fact that men and women are different. They explain that when God created Adam, Eve had not been created yet. On the other hand, when God created Eve, Adam was asleep. Hence Adam did not know how Eve was created, while Eve had no clear idea about how Adam came into existence. Therefore, neither of them knew the other.

Birth

The difference becomes evident immediately, when at the maternity ward a woman gives birth. To begin with, the Midwife takes the child immediately after delivery, raises it up and says, "it is a boy" or "it is a girl". The sex of the child is apparent because of their sexual organs – Penis for the boy and vagina for the girl. This is the real difference between a man and a woman. When they grow up during the teenage years, there are complicated changes. The boy, during puberty, develops a low voice. His nipples remain the same but he develops hair around the face, pubic area and armpits and also starts producing sperm. The girl goes through a very complex biological process involving the enlargement of the breasts and hips, the appearance of pubic and underarm hair and the arrival of a monthly menstrual cycle. These differences between the man and woman are crucial in their lives and naturally affect their relationship.

Apart from the sex organs and other obvious physical differences, there are other important differences such as the emotions, psychological make-up, thought processes and memory.

God in His infinite wisdom made men and women different in order for them to play complementary roles and to use the differences to strengthen their partnership.

Relationships between men and women are not necessarily difficult. Problems arise when we expect or assume the opposite sex should think, feel or act the same way we do. As stated by T.D Jakes, "What makes life interesting, what makes a conversation stimulating is people with differing points of view. Those who need others to think and act exactly the way they do are often masking insecurities, and have a deep-seated need to have their views and actions confirmed in the behaviour and thought of others. Disagreements happen in any relationship where more than one person is involved; it's inevitable"

However, our attitude and the way we approach the

disagreements makes the difference.

Therefore, if you want to build and sustain a lasting relationship, the secret is to acknowledge that differences exist. This knowledge will prevent you from building your relationship on a weak foundation. It is the lack of knowledge and experience which leads to difficulties, challenges and problems.

A friend sent us a joke on Facebook. It is entitled, the difference between a man and a woman. This was adapted from Jokes.com. Kindly read and smile:

1. A woman worries about the future until she gets a husband. A man never worries about the future until he gets a wife.

2. A successful man is one who makes more money than his wife can spend. A successful woman is one who can find such a man.

3. To be happy with a man, you must understand him a lot & love him a little. To be happy with a woman, you must love her a lot & not try to understand her at all.

4. Married men live longer than single men – but married men are a lot more willing to die.

5. Any married man should forget his mistakes – there's no use in two people remembering the same thing.

6. Men wake up as good-looking as they went to bed. Women somehow deteriorate during the night.

7. A woman marries a man expecting he will change, but he doesn't. A man marries a woman expecting that she won't change & she does.

8. A woman has the last word in any argument. Anything a man says after that is the beginning of a new argument.

9. There are 2 times when a man doesn't understand a woman - before marriage & after marriage.

We love stories and we love to share the relevant ones especially when the are related to what we are writing about. And so here we go. A lady friend sent us this information via email. Please read on. It is entitled, *the woman God created*;

When God created woman, He was working late on the 6th day.

An Angel came by and said: "Why spend so much time on that one?"

And the Lord answered: "Have you seen all the specifications I have to meet to shape her?"

"She must be washable, but not made of plastic, have more than 200 moving parts which must all be replaceable and she must function on all kinds of food. She must be able to embrace several kids at the same time, give a hug that can heal anything from a bruised knee to a broken heart and she must do all this with only two hands".

The Angel was impressed. "Just two hands... impossible". And this is the standard model?!

"Too much work for one day ... Wait until tomorrow and then complete her".

"I will not "said the Lord. I am so close to completing this creation, which will be the favourite of my heart".

The Lord continued "She cures herself when sick and she can work 18 hours a day".

The Angel came nearer and touched this woman.

"But you have made her soft Lord"

"She is soft" said the Lord, "But I have also made her strong. You can't imagine what she can endure and overcome".

"Can she think?" The angel asked.

"Not only can she think, she can reason and negotiate".

The Angel touched the woman's cheek…

"Lord it seems this creation is leaking! You have put too many burdens on her".

She is not leaking…it's a tear. The Lord corrected the Angel.

"What is it for?" asked the Angel.

And the Lord said: "Tears are her way of expressing grief, her doubts, her love, her loneliness, her suffering, and her pride!"

This made a big impression on the Angel. "Lord you are a genius. You thought of everything, the woman is indeed marvellous!"

Indeed she is!

Woman has strengths that amaze man. She can handle trouble and carry heavy burdens.

She holds happiness, love and opinions. She smiles when feeling like screaming. She sings when she feels like crying, cries when she is happy and laughs when she is afraid.

She fights for what she believes in and stands up against injustice.

She doesn't take "no" for an answer. When she can see a better solution, she gives herself so her family can thrive. She takes her friend to the Doctor if she is afraid. Her love is unconditional.

She cries when her kids are victorious. She is happy when her friends do well. She is glad when she hears of a birth or a wedding.

Her heart is broken when a next of kin or friend dies.

But she finds the strength to get on with life.

She knows that a kiss and a hug can heal a broken heart.

There is only one thing wrong with her.

She forgets her worth.

NB; Tell this to your lady friends to remind them how fantastic they are. Tell it to the males you know. Sometimes, they need to be reminded.

H/C

CONCLUSION

It is a well-known fact that marriage does not enjoy very good public relations. Even among Christians, the statistics are frightening. With almost about 50% marriages collapsing within the first five years, the need to find a solution has never been urgent.

But the root cause as stated above can be traced to the issue of choice. When people make choices based on what the media is saying or by worldly standards instead of the laid down biblical principles or the word of God, there is bound to be problems. It is important for singles to know that choosing a partner for marriage is about the future. It is not about the now. Since one does not know the future, he or she should stick to what the word of God says. This will guarantee you a better foundation.

The important thing about courtship is the time it enables you to spend together with your mate; to study each other, ask questions and get the necessary clarifications about issues. Courtship is not marriage and therefore you should not throw caution to the wind. However, if this opportunity is missed because you think you can now break your set boundaries and start indulging in sex among others, then you are in for future disappointment.

We have had the opportunity to counsel several individuals before they finally ended up at the altar. Though counsellors cannot play God by advising against certain relationships, it is important that individuals in love do their homework well before finally sealing their relationship. Yes you may be in love. That is fine. But you need more than love start a marriage and to sustain it.

Divorce is real. Therefore, it is important that you take pre-marital counselling seriously. Unfortunately, most Christian partners are sometimes more focused on going through the training with the view to getting the approval of their Pastors.

It is our considered opinion that pre-marital counselling should be made compulsory in the Churches. Those Churches that do not have qualified or trained Christian Counsellors should contract others to help train some of their members. There are several wounded people in the Church due to marital break downs and disappointments. The emotional pains that follow sometimes become permanent scars and detrimentally affect the person's future. This can be resolved through getting the Counsellors in place.

The Bible says that 'for lack of knowledge my people perish.' Knowledge about God's honourable institution will bring you the essential foundations for your marriage. Therefore, if you follow the valuable advice provided in this book, we can guarantee to a greater extent that your marriage will work.

We wish you all the best in your reading. Do not stop educating yourself about how to make your marriage sustainable. When you need help, information, advise and guidance i.e. counselling or talking to someone about specific issues, The House of change and other Christian counsellors are available to help you.

To your success. God bless you.

Bibliography

- Aris Sharon: Being Married. Your guide to a happy modern marriage. Australia, 2004

- Collins Gary: Christian Counselling. A comprehensive guide. Cheltenham. 2007

- Dobson James Dr.: What wives wish their husbands knew about women.USA.1985

- Goerz, Allan and Donna: A Pre-marriage Counselling Handbook, Challenge Enterprise of Ghana, 2004

- Jakes, TD; Before You Do. Making great decisions that you won't regret.2008

- Litvinoff Sarah: The relate guide to better relationships. Practical ways to make your love last. London 1998

- Munroe Myles Dr: Single, Married, Separated, & Life After Divorce. USA. 2003

- Munroe Myles Dr: Waiting and Dating. A sensible guide to fulfilling love relationships. USA, 2004

- Persaud Raj Dr.:Simply Irresistible. The Psychology of Seduction. How to catch and keep your perfect partner. London 2006

- Waines Alison: Making Relationships Work. Great Britain, 2005

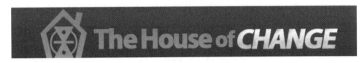

ORDER FORM

If you would like to order copies of this book, please complete this order form and send it to the address below:

Name _____

Address: _____

_____

Tel: _____

Email _____

Number of copies: _____

Please send a £11.97 cheque, postal or money order for one book purchase. Postage and delivery is inclusive. Book will be dispatched immediately payment is received at the bank or post office.

We provide special rates and free shipment to Churches and book stores who buy in bulk

Please address your request to:
William Appiah
The House of Change
Unit 7 Excalibur Works
13 Argall Avenue
Argall Industrial Estates
E10 7QE, London, UK

Here's A Special Bonus

As a special bonus with your purchase or opt in with your email address today, you will also receive a monthly newsletter and emails on relationships and our products.

Please take a look at the membership subscription for EITHER

Christian Singles Relationship Lessons (Courtship) : http://thehouseofchange.com/ChristianSinglesRelationship/

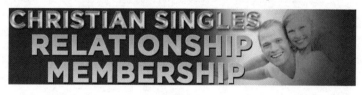

OR

Dating Christian Singles Lessons : http://thehouseofchange.com/DatingChristianSingles/

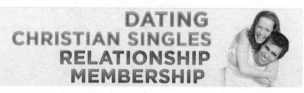

Where we provide exclusive lessons, information and advice to members and subscribers on how to build and sustain their relationship towards marriage.

WOMEN ISSUES

Please Visit The Following Website To Discover More Information On Women Empowerment Issues;

http://www.MinisterDorothyMinistries.com

ATTENTION AFRICAN PASTORS WIVES
JOIN SAFERHAVEN

Safer Haven is a place of support in confidence, for wives of African Pastors Worldwide. SaferHaven is committed to providing a sanctuary for wives and aspiring wives of African Pastors worldwide. We promote knowledge, skills, and insights using a personal and professional approach based on the Bible as the inspired Word of God. We focus on practical ways to develop the skills, knowledge and understanding of wives of African Pastors worldwide to support their husbands' in their ministry.

We Provide support to wives and wives-to-be of African Pastors in their daily challenges of living, emphasising on what they can do to change the situation, build their ministry and live a God fulfilled life.

Visit The Following Website To Discover More Information On African Pastors Wives Issues; http://www.saferhaven. com

1-ON-1 COACHING

Successful Real Lasting Change Guaranteed if You Join The...

EXCLUSIVE 1-ON-1 PERSONNAL DEVELOPMENT AND LIFE BREAKTHROUGH COACHING PROGRAMME, ONCE A WEEK WITH WILLAM & REV. MRS DOROTHY APPIAH

VIA

 OR **+**

FROM THE LUXURY OF YOUR HOME
If you are looking for a Christian Coach to help you achieve your goal on weekly basis, then read on.

Who Is This Coaching Programme For?

This Coaching programme has been created specifically for **Christians who have a personal desire to achieve their goals and need both a road map and a good tour guide in the process.**

For More Information, please go to WWW. TheHouseOfChange.com

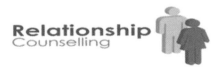

Top Secrets to Be Revealed! Excellent Group Lessons to Help You...

ENJOY YOUR DATING, COURTSHIP AND OR PRE-MARITAL LESSONS (1ST & SUBSEQUENT MARRIAGES) TWICE A WEEK, FOR SIX WEEKS, WITH **WILLIAM AND REV. DOROTHY APPIAH** IN THE COMFORT OF YOUR HOME

VIA

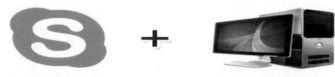

- Are you new in your relationship or thinking of entering into a fresh one?
- Are you currently facing problems in your relationship, i.e. Dating and Courtship and need lessons, advice and guidance? Don't throw in the towel yet. It does not matter the current state of your relationship. With God all things are possible.
- Are you single? Do you have some specific issues that you need to be educated, informed or advised on?
- Are thinking of getting into a second marriage?
- Are you about to get married and need a Christian Pre-marriage Lessons to help you through the journey with guaranteed results, Before You Say "I Do"?

THEN JOIN THE 6-WEEK GROUP COURSE FOR SINGLES, DATING& PRE-MARITAL INDIVIDUALS.
For More Information, please go to WWW.TheHouseOfChange.com

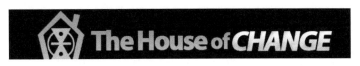

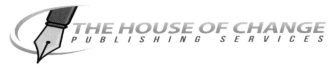

Ready To Get Your Book Published In 40 Days Or Less?

If you want to get your book published professionally in paperback, we can do all the hard work for you; promote, market and distribute your book through various platforms including Amazon.com, Ingram, Barnes and Noble and other reputable book giants. We would help to make your title available to more than 39,000 retailers and libraries worldwide and therefore guarantee access to more readers across the world.

We will also help to distribute your book via Smashwords to major online retailers such as Apple (distribution to iBooks stores in 51 countries), Barnes & Noble (US and UK), Scribd, Oyster, Kobo, OverDrive (world's largest library ebook platform serving 20,000+ libraries), Flipkart: India's largest online bookseller), Baker & Taylor (Blio and the Axis360 library service), Page Foundry (operates retail sites Inktera.com and Versent.com; and operates Android ebook store apps for Cricket Wireless and Asus), and other distribution outlets.

We take away the hassle of guess work and problems associated with self-publishing. What is more, you will get professional help from us in addition to maintaining 100% of your publishing rights and 100% of your profits.

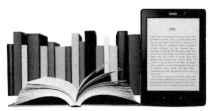

FOR MORE INFORMATION, GO TO

http://thehouseofchange.com/book_publishing/index.html

RECOMMENDED eBOOKS FROM OUR BOOKSTORE

THE FOLLOWING BEST-SELLING eBOOKS CO-AUTHORED BY US ARE HIGHLY RECOMMENDED.

FUNNY STORIES AND JOKES FOR YOUR RELATIONSHIP

Humorous Stories And Jokes To Spice Up Relationships And Marriages

Price: $9.97

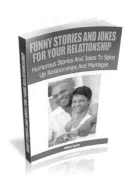

FUNNY STORIES AND JOKES FOR WOMEN

Humorous Stories And Jokes To Spice Up Relationships

Price: $9.97

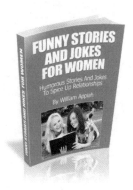

BE INSPIRED FOR DAILY LIVING

Short Stories And Inspirational Words To Spice Up Your Daily Life

$9.97

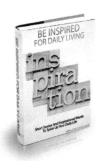

And So He Laughed Her Head Off

Humorous Stories And Jokes To Spice Up Relationships and Marriages

Price: $9.97

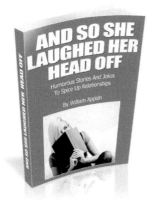

Misunderstanding In The Relationship

How To Deal With This "Little Fox" In Your Relationship

FREE

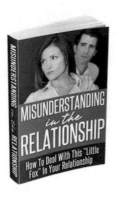

Arguments and Disagreements In The Relationship

How To Deal With These Two "Little Foxes" In Your Relationship

FREE

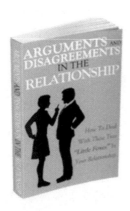

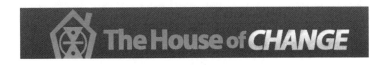

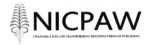

NETWORK OF INDEPENDENT CHRISTIAN PUBLISH-ERS AND WRITERS (NiCPAW)

We destroy arguments and every proud obstacle to the knowl-edge of God, and take every thought captive to obey Christ, 2 Corinthians 10:5

NICPAW provide information, education and training as well as resources and opportunities for every Christian involved in or interested in publishing, such as writers, authors, freelance writers, publishers and artists.

NICPAW also encourages networking through the exchange of ideas, information, and other mutual benefits including being a member of our exclusive Facebook group.

Join Our Membership Now

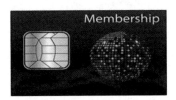

FOR MORE INFORMATION:

Email: NICPAW@TheHouseOfChange.com/network
Website: www.TheHouseOfChange.com/network

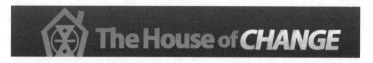

CHECK OUR WEBSITE FOR MORE INFORMATION AND RESOURCES ABOUT OUR PRODUCTS:

- CDs
- DVDs
- eBooks
- Physical Books
- Home Study Relationship Programmes
- Church Training and Capacity Building Programmes
- Church Package
- Membership (Dating and Courtship)
- Relationship Master Class
- Magazine
- Newsletter
- Public Speaking Programmes
- Events and Seminars
- Webinars
- Book Publishing
- Network of Independent Christian Publishers and Writers
- Affiliate (Earn a Commission) Programme

Check Our Website: www.TheHouseOfChange.com

BUY NOW FROM OUR WEBSITE OR AMAZON.COM

Please leave a comment after purchase

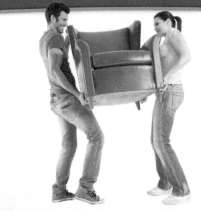